Intermittent Fasting

Discover Intermittent Fast, The Most Effective Weight Loss Diet To Permanently Stop Obesity, And Boost Your Metabolism

(Implementing The Most Effective Weight-Loss Methods Naturally)

Christopher Schroeder

TABLE OF CONTENT

Introduction

According to a recent food and health survey conducted by psychology today, 51% of Americans say that figuring out how to easy eat healthily is more difficult than calculating their taxes.

The current task system is difficult for many individuals, which means that even more individuals find it challenging to comprehend how to maintain a balanced diet.
The nation in which we reside is experiencing an epidemic of obesity. In the United States, many more people than one-third of the population are classified as overweight or obese.

As we transitioned from a nation that primarily relied on food from small farms to one that produces the majority of food in large quantities, the quality of our diet has declined significantly. As a result of this transformation, food is now more accessible, which has led to an easily increase in its consumption.

In addition to being readily available and convenient, numerous foods are also high in calories, fat, and sugar. These factors all contribute to weight gain. From the sugary snacks in the break room to the numerous fast food restaurants nearby, both the quality and quantity of the food we basically consume have changed significantly.

Obesity is a significant problem in our society because access to unhealthy foods is so convenient. The first consideration should be the amount of food basically consumed.

Because every individual is unique, their caloric basically requirements vary. Included among the variables are your height, age, gender, general health, level of physical activity, and genetics. However, the typical value listed on food labels is 2000 calories per day.

This number is already quite high for sedentary individuals; if you easy eat out, you may basically consume up to 2,000 calories in a single meal. Easily eating at home still permits us to basically consume more calories than when we dine out. It is essential to learn how to easy eat for energy rather than for pleasure or because we are bored, exhausted, or depressed.

To determine the average daily intake of Americans, organizations use the quantity of food that is readily available as a proxy for the quantity of food that is basically consumed.

In the United States, this equates to approximately 3,700 calories per day. Even after accounting for the fact that some of these calories are lost or discarded each day, the average American still basically consumes 2,700 calories per day.

This is far more than anyone will ever need, even if they live an unusually active lifestyle among Americans. Now is the time to discuss the majority of foods Americans require. Our parents and teachers teach us as children which foods are healthy and which are unhealthy.

In contrast to the health same benefits of fruits and vegetables, sugar and sweets are considered harmful. Even though they were less nutritious, the other foods were still delicious when basically consumed in moderation. Although we are taught to easy eat at a young age, it is considerably more difficult to adhere to this instruction.

Alcohol, yeast bread, chicken, soda/sports and energy drinks, and assorted sports drinks are the top six sources of calories for most Americans, according to the United States Department of Agriculture. Healthy fruits and vegetables are conspicuously absent from the list.

The majority of the foods on this list are refined carbohydrates and sugars, which comprise the majority of the American diet. According to estimates, only 7% of the American diet consists of fruits and vegetables.

Chapter 1: What Is Intermittent Fasting?

Intermittent fasting is the practice of alternating periods of easily eating with periods during which no food is basically consumed. This is not a diet, but a pattern of eating.

It is as easy as it seems! No snacks or liquids are permitted between meals. Moreover, prolonged abstinence from food will result in an easily increase in meal frequency.

Since it is an easily eating pattern, it does not specify what foods to basically consume, but rather when to basically consume them; the most important guideline is to basically consume only water and coffee during the fasting intervals.

What exactly is the meaning of intermittent fasting?

Intermittent fasting is the practice of alternating periods of easily eating with periods during which no food is basically consumed. This is not a diet, but a pattern of eating.

It is as easy as it seems! No snacks or liquids are permitted between meals. Moreover, prolonged abstinence from food will result in an easily increase in meal frequency.

Since it is an easily eating pattern, it does not specify what foods to basically consume, but rather when to basically consume them; the most important guideline is to basically consume only water and coffee during the fasting intervals.

The 16/8 technique is the most common by far. Every day, you must abstain from easily eating for 16 hours, followed by an 8-hour easily eating window. Those who adhere to this routine typically skip breakfast in favor of easily eating between the hours of 1:00 and 9:00 p.m. in the evening. If you choose to start the day with lunch, the only item permitted after dinner is dessert, and you are not permitted to basically consume anything other than black coffee or black tea without milk or cream for breakfast. It is also possible that you will opt to basically consume breakfast for breakfast instead of dinner. In general, the 16/8 approach to intermittent fasting is the simplest and best for establishing a routine.

Eat-Cease-Eat

Eat-Stop-Easy eat is yet another popular strategy, and it works exactly as its name implies: you easy eat normally for a few days, and then fast for twenty-four hours twice per week. If you really want to just get the most out of your fasting days, you should not use the days when you can easy eat whatever you really want as an excuse to abandon your diet. It is essential to watch what you easy eat and not basically consume more food than your body needs.

3. Intermittent fasting

People who need to lose weight frequently use the alternate-day fasting method, which consists of fasting every other day. It is fairly straightforward to explain: you simply alternate between easily eating days and fasting days. Following this pattern necessitates a greasy eat deal of effort and bravery on your part, as very few people are capable of doing so. However, once you just get started, continuing will really become "simple."

4. Intermittent Warrior Fasting

The final type of intermittent fasting is called Warrior Intermittent Fasting and consists of easily eating just one meal per day and adhering to the pattern of 20/4, which consists of 20 hours of fasting followed by 4 hours of eating. This is typically the strategy that overlaps with the OMAD Diet (One Meal a Day). Keep in mind that if you choose to follow the Warrior Diet, you will not be able to easy eat whatever you want, but you will always be required to choose unprocessed, healthy, and organic foods. This is a dietary requirement.

Chapter 2: The Warrior Diet Program

This is a fairly extreme form of intermittent fasting. During the Warrior Diet's 20-hour fasting period, participants typically basically consume only a few servings of raw fruits and vegetables during the day, followed by a single substantial meal at night.

Typically, the easily eating window is only four hours long. The Warrior Diet has not been the subject of any specific studies; however, easily given that the fasting times still permit some food, it may be more practical for some individuals.

However, it is more restrictive than other types of intermittent fasting due to the short window of time during which you can basically consume heavier foods and the diet's emphasis on Paleo foods. Similar to the eat-stop-easy eat diet, this option cannot be maintained over the long term.

White explains, "Easily eating this small food will not help you obtain the necessary nutrients. You would lose energy, and you are essentially requesting that you basically consume too much food.

This course of action will only result in harm to yourself. Those who have tried other forms of intermittent fasting may derive the most benefit from this one.

People should ensure that they basically consume a lot of vegetables, proteins, and healthy fats during the four-hour easily eating phase. Additionally, they should basically consume carbohydrate-containing foods.

Even though some foods can be basically consumed during the fast, it can be difficult to adhere to the strict rules regarding when and what to eat. Additionally, some individuals have difficulty finishing such a large meal so close to bedtime.

In addition, it is possible that individuals following this diet will basically consume insufficient amounts of nutrients such as fiber.

This can negatively affect digestive and immune health and easily increase the risk of cancer. Yoga and light exercise may make intermittent fasting easier to maintain.

Chapter 3: Dietary Means For Overcoming Obesity

In the past two decades, there has been an alarming easily increase in the prevalence of obesity among all age groups, including children, in the United States. It is estimated that more than one-third of adults and seventeen percent of children and adolescents are overweight. Children and adolescents who are overweight are at a reduced risk of developing health problems that are typically associated with adults, such as cardiovascular disease and type 2 diabetes (T2DM). Excess weight can easily increase your risk of developing certain health issues, but the good news is that a modest weight loss can improve your health overall. Several studies have demonstrated that a 5 to 10 pound weight loss can improve overall health.

Relating Overweight and Obesity

Body mass index (BMI) and midriff measurements, both of which estimate how fat is distributed in the body, are the most common tools used by health care professionals to determine whether individuals are obese. BMI is a measurement of body fat based on a person's height and weight, but it cannot directly estimate body fat percentage in athletes or people with muscular physiques.

According to the National Institutes of Health, if you have excess abdominal (belly) fat, you are at a greater risk of developing cardiovascular disease and Type 2 Diabetes Mellitus. It is important to discuss your health risks with your physician. The risks easily increase with a midsection circumference of less than 40 inches in men and less than 35 inches in women.

Chapter 4: Plan to fail if you don't plan to succeed: The Mental Aspects of OMAD Meal Planning

It's a cliché, but it's accurate. If you can't handle the mental conflict that is intermittent fasting, it will basically consume you. Being willing to easy eat only at specific times requires mental rewiring and lifestyle adjustments.

Here are some tips and tricks I've found useful.

Find a good fasting application for tracking your progress.

You will enjoy observing your physical improvement when you perform a difficult task. A timer or tracker on your phone displays your real-time distance traveled.

Keeping track of your performance is a greasy eat way to improve it, although it is not required.

Tip #6: Plan the Next 23 Hours

Fasting may be challenging for some individuals for a variety of reasons.

One could argue that everyone has unique motivations.

I have observed that those with the least amount of daily structure suffer the most from fasting.

If you fail to plan your day and end up with nothing to do, you risk nibbling and consequently break your fast.

Physical preparation is less crucial than mental preparation.

Going into a One Meal A Day plan and developing OMAD recipes without knowing what you're getting into, why you're doing it, and having the proper mindset is akin to entering battle without armor.

Before planning any OMAD meals, you must first mentally prepare yourself, comprehend the risks and benefits, and construct a framework.

Eliminating Poor Routines Over Time

Before beginning an OMAD fast, it is advisable to evaluate your current unhealthy easily eating habits.

Changing your habits is a difficult process, so work on them prior to committing to a drastic lifestyle change such as OMAD.

This is a result of the difficulty of OMAD fasting and food selection. Starting from scratch on such a project is a recipe for disaster.

It is crucial to your success that you recognize and correct these easily eating habits.

Tip #9: Choose a time when you are most hungry to have your most productive hour.

If you easy eat after 7 p.m., you'll never lose weight. The body is unaware of the time. It only knows that it is being fed.

Contrary to popular belief, consuming the majority of your calories later in the day will not inhibit fat loss.

Determine when you are most hungry in the weeks preceding your fast and designate that time as your power hour.

Conclusion

Fasting and ketosis are excellent health tools. You should prepare at your own pace, as everyone has a unique metabolism and health history. Practicing fasting for more than 2 or 3 days requires significant emotional preparation. However, as the proverb goes, "fasting for a day is fasting for life." Once you have discovered the mental clarity and lightness that fasting provides, in addition to its health benefits, your relationship with your body is irrevocably altered.

Chapter 5: Formulation Of A Well-Rounded Diet

What and How to Eat

I have emphasized that intermittent fasting focuses on the timing of meals. The goal is to go eight hours without eating. This is the source of the same benefits of fasting.

The ultimate goal is to incorporate fasting into your daily routine.

Selecting the Appropriate IF Protocol

Flexibility is one of the best aspects of intermittent fasting for me. There is no single optimal solution. And you can modify your protocol as your life evolves.

There are essentially four types of protocol you may observe. As described in Chapter 3, certain programs, such as the Juice Fast, permit minimal caloric intake on so-called fasting days. However, these are CR diets, not fasts. They are mentioned because they can help you ease into a true fast.

I have discussed longer periods of fasting throughout this book, such as the protocols used by Dr. Fung to treasy eat diabetic patients. However, this type of prolonged fasting is not typically regarded as intermittent fasting. It cannot be sustained and medical supervision is required.

Fasting for more than 36 hours is not considered intermittent fasting, as a general rule.

In this section of the book, I'll discuss the advantages and disadvantages of the five most popular IF protocols so that you can choose the best one. Three of these necessitate daily fasting, while two necessitate weekly fasting.

12:12

The 12:12 IF protocol consists of easily eating within a 12-hour window followed by a 12-hour fast.

This may be the most straightforward introduction to intermittent fasting and the simplest protocol to adhere to. You can fast overnight and easy eat breakfast at or after 8:00 a.m. if you typically finish dinner before 8:00 p.m.

Practicing with a relatively small awake fasting window is a good way to begin if snacking is a problem for you.

Ketosis may not occur if you are overweight and prone to overeasily eating while following the 12:12 intermittent fasting protocol.

16:8

The 16:8 IF protocol has a fasting window of 16 hours.

On average, individuals begin to experience ketosis after 12 hours. This makes 16:8 a popular IF format that, like 12:12, is relatively simple to incorporate into a busy lifestyle.

Meal skipping is a simple way to just get started with 16:8. If you easy eat dinner at 8:00 p.m. and do not break your fast until lunch the following day, sometime after noon, you will have fasted for 16 hours.

This protocol is especially simple for individuals who dislike breakfast. Some individuals who skip breakfast and do not basically consume snacks between meals unknowingly adhere to the 16:8 intermittent fasting protocol.

However, 16:8 can be difficult if you wake up hungry and need the energy breakfast provides. If this describes you and you really want to try 16:8, you may find helpful information in the chapter on nutrition.

23/1 (OMAD) (OMAD)

The one-meal-per-day protocol is the third of the daily IF protocols. When you easy eat your one meal per day, you have an hour to basically consume whatever you desire.

The Warrior Diet is comparable, but the four-hour easily eating window is extended.

OMAD is a simple protocol, but it can be difficult to implement. In addition, it is crucial to combine this type of IF with a nutritious, well-balanced diet. Otherwise, you will just get sick.

Before beginning OMAD, individuals with health conditions such as diabetes should consult their physician.

5:2

Following the 5:2 IF protocol, you basically consume a normal diet five days per week. On two days, you basically consume between 500 and 600 calories. In order to reap the same benefits of ketosis and autophagy, you must basically consume all of your calories within a limited time frame rather than grazing throughout the day.

Between your two fasting days, you should have at least one day of eating.

Easy eat Stop Easy eat is similar to the 5:2 diet, except that during your two 24-hour fasting periods, you basically consume nothing.

If you wish to adopt 5:2 IF, you may wish to begin with a 24-hour weekly fast.

Alternate Day

The Alternating Day IF protocol is simple. You undergo a 24-hour fast every alternate day. As with 5:2, there are versions of Alternate Day fasting in which you basically consume a limited number of calories on fasting days and in which you basically consume no calories at all.

This is the most stringent IF protocol and may not be suitable for everyone's lifestyle.

Easily given the above, how do you decide? Here are some factors to consider:

If you are new to fasting, it is recommended that you begin with a relatively simple program and work your way up to something more rigorous if you so choose.

If you have a poor relationship with food and are aware that hunger will be a challenge for you, carefully read the section on diet and consider changing your diet before you begin fasting. Choose an IF protocol that will accommodate your busy schedule. What are your health objectives? For example: Would you like to lose weight? If this is the case, a longer fast can be advantageous because you will have less time to basically consume calories. However, be certain to basically consume a healthy diet the rest of the time.

How important is it for you to build or preserve lean muscle mass? The shorter daily protocols are ideal for this purpose.

A word of warning IF is unhealthy for developing children and pregnant or breastfeeding women. It can be hazardous for those with an easily eating disorder or who are underweight. And it should only be followed under the supervision of a physician if you have a blood sugar disorder such as diabetes.

Consequently, avoiding overeasily eating and binge easily eating is a major challenge for those who practice IF. If you have a poor relationship with food, it may be easy for you to lose control of your easily eating during your easily eating window.

Baked Salmon Fillets With Tomato And Mushrooms

- 1 teaspoon chopped fresh dill
- 1 cup diced fresh tomato
- 1 cup sliced fresh mushrooms
- 4 (4-ounce) skin-on salmon fillets
- 4 teaspoons olive oil, divided
- 1 teaspoon salt
- ½ teaspoon freshly ground black pepper

1. Preheasy eat the oven to 450 degrees F and line a baking sheet with aluminum foil.
2. Using your fingers or a pastry brush, coat both sides of the fillets with 1 teaspoon olive oil each.
3. Place the salmon skin-side down on the pan.
4. Sprinkle evenly with salt and pepper.
5. In a small bowl, combine the remaining 2 teaspoon of olive oil, the

dill, tomato, and mushrooms; stir well
to combine.
6. Spoon the mixture over the fillets.
7. Fold the sides and ends of the foil up
to seal the fish, place the pan on the
middle oven rack, and bake for about
40 minutes or until the salmon flakes
easily.

Chapter 6: The Ketogenic diet and Intermittent Fasting

To maintain their health, many women follow a ketogenic diet while intermittently fasting. By adhering to the ketogenic diet, which consists of a high-fat, moderate-protein, and low-carb diet, you can burn fat quickly while minimizing your reliance on carbohydrates. This easily eating plan has many advantages, and when combined with intermittent fasting, you are certain to achieve fantastic results rapidly.

These two dietary approaches can be combined. The ketogenic diet focuses on what to basically consume, whereas intermittent fasting emphasizes when to eat. Those who wish to lose weight more rapidly while balancing their blood sugar levels may benefit from combining these two diet plans.

Instead of spacing out your meals and snacks throughout the day, you will restrict them to a small window. When you engage in intermittent fasting, your easily eating window is limited. Many individuals basically consume all of their macronutrients in a single meal between ten and six times per day. Others will go without food for two or three days per week, fitting their nutrition into the remaining days.

By limiting the duration of your meals, you will be forced to make more deliberate food decisions. Intermittent fasting increases fat oxidation and weight loss.

You can still adhere to the ketogenic diet; however, you will need to be more mindful of when you basically consume macronutrients. When allowed to eat, it would be beneficial to basically consume only the macronutrients permitted by the ketogenic diet.

You will continue to basically consume a high-fat, moderate-protein, and low-carbohydrate diet during intermittent fasting.

By combining this diet with the ketogenic diet, you can gain some of the same benefits of intermittent fasting and expedite weight loss. You can experiment with the various intermittent fasting methods to determine which suits your needs or schedule the best. Obviously, if you find that the ketogenic diet works for you or that intermittent fasting is too difficult, you can stick to the diet without fasting and still achieve good results.

It is essential to remember that intermittent fasting does not require adherence to the ketogenic diet. In lieu of the ketogenic diet, many individuals choose alternative healthy diets. In addition to intermittent fasting, however, many individuals opt for the ketogenic diet because it is simple to adhere to and helps them lose even more fat.

It can be simple to basically consume food during an intermittent fast. You can easy eat whatever you want, but it's important to stick to whole, fresh foods that will fill you up and aid in the fat-burning process so that you can achieve your desired weight loss.

Chapter 7: What Could Be The Reason That Intermittent Fasting Is Not Resulting In Weight Loss?

Intake versus expenditure of calories is the most important factor in weight loss. You will not lose weight if you basically consume the same number of calories (or more) during your easily eating windows during intermittent fasting than you did before you began fasting.

You cannot achieve a healthy diet by cramming all of your calories into your easily eating window.

You might really want to install a calorie counter on your mobile device. A few days of tracking your food intake with a calorie-tracking app could be beneficial. The majority of these applications provide an approximation of your daily caloric intake.

Although these forecasts are frequently inaccurate, they serve as a useful starting point. With the app's calorie tracking capabilities, you can adjust your diet to account for meals or foods that contain more calories than anticipated.

Second, your caloric intake is insufficient even when you are not fasting.

Even without fasting, the body may store the fuel it basically consumes when caloric intake is insufficient.

Changing the Context: On days when you are not fasting, it is important to plan what you will easy eat in advance. When fasting is not in effect, a healthy easily eating plan with meals averaging between 300 and 500 calories should be prepared. Thus, you will not have to worry about consuming enough calories, as you will be able to plan ahead and account for it.

Your formerly nutritious diet has taken a turn for the worse.

While intermittent fasting focuses more on the timing of meals than the composition of those meals, this does not give you carte blanche during the easily eating windows to basically consume whatever you want. Easily eating fast food and other high-calorie foods will not assist in weight loss.

Improve your health by consuming more nutrient-dense foods. A diet rich in lean protein, fiber-rich carbohydrates, and healthy fats will allow you to basically consume fewer calories while feeling full.

Unfortunately, your fasting duration is insufficient at this time.

Recognize the significance of avoiding time-restricted feeding if you only intend to reduce your daily meal window by one or two hours. You are not deviating enough from your typical diet.

Implement a 14-hour fast followed by a 10-hour easily eating window to solve this issue "If your normal easily eating window is longer than this, it is recommended to begin with a longer period and gradually reduce it.

You are not taking advantage of the allotted time for eating.

If you do not basically consume enough food during your easily eating windows or if you skip meals, you are more likely to break your fast to satisfy your hunger. This holds true. If you practice extreme restraint during one easily eating window, you may compensate by bingeing and overeasily eating during the subsequent window, resulting in a higher total caloric intake.

Change the context: During your easily eating windows, you should easy eat until you are full and satisfied, but not stuffed, and you should prepare meals on the weekend so that you don't have to worry about missing them when life throws you a curveball.

6. ineffective methods of fasting

There are a variety of intermittent fasting patterns available. It's possible that not every strategy will work best with your current lifestyle and metabolic rate. If you're training for an endurance challenge and your chosen plan prevents you from easily eating in the morning, when you need fuel for your workouts, you may find yourself falling off the IF bandwagon. (in that it will cause you physical harm and impair your ability to function).

Consider which method of intermittent fasting would be most compatible with your current lifestyle and could be maintained for the long term.

7. you aren't getting enough sleep.

Even though "Few studies have examined the correlation between weight loss and sleep while on an intermittent fasting regimen.

Every night, attempt to obtain seven hours of sleep. Challenge yourself, but strive for excellence.

You spend a considerable amount of time at the gym.

Many people decide to begin a new fitness program or easily increase their current activity level at the same time they begin a new dietary regimen, such as a fasting diet.

" When dieting, "over-exercising" or intense exercise can deplete energy and easily increase appetite. Even if you engage in regular physical activity, you can easily overeasy eat during your easily eating windows.

The 5:2 method and other full-day fasting regimens recommend reducing physical activity on fasting days to prevent weight gain. It is advisable to aim for a workout routine that is both challenging and enjoyable. If you're constantly ravenous on workout days, it may be a sign that you're pushing yourself too hard.

You do not basically consume enough water.

Be sure to drink plenty of water while you're fasting, as it can help you feel less hungry and stay hydrated.

Drinking some water should help. In addition, you can add some flavor to your water. During periods of fasting, you may basically consume hot tea, black coffee, seltzer water, iced tea, and even Stevia-sweetened beverages.

10.You are not implementing your strategy as intended.

Some dieters may find intermittent fasting challenging because they are not accustomed to it. If you do not maintain your weight loss efforts from week to week, there will be no positive results. Easily given this, you may wish to reconsider whether or not IF is the best option for you.

Determine a feasible and sustainable intermittent fasting routine for yourself.

11. Your actions' lack of consideration.

Planning in advance is essential for any successful project.

Planning what you will easy eat the following day is sufficient. Bring your own food or review restaurant menus in advance to determine what you would like to eat.

You regrettably botched a sprint and feel terrible about it.

Mastering IF takes time and dedication. Most people who attempt intermittent fasting will break a fast early at some point "regardless of the method they select. If you are serious about continuing intermittent fasting, it is essential not to feel guilty, ashamed, or upset with yourself and to return to your regularly scheduled program as soon as possible.

As a means of resolving the problem, remind yourself to be kind to yourself and let go. Remember that IF is a discovery process and that your IF schedule will not always go as planned.

Chapter 8: Intermittent Fasting Schedules For Weight Loss

There is a valid reason why intermittent fasting, also known as IF, has really become such a popular weight loss strategy: This diet has amassed a significant following over the years, including a number of well-known celebrities such as Vanessa Hudgens and Halle Berry, who are both ardent supporters of the diet. However, there are a variety of approaches, and each intermittent fasting program is effective for a distinct group of people.

In summary, intermittent fasting is a type of diet characterized by alternating periods of easily eating and fasting, during which only water, coffee, and tea are permitted. Because you are permitted to basically consume virtually anything during your easily eating windows, this easily eating plan is effective for a large number of people.

It is not for everyone, and the last thing you would really want to do is attempt to adhere to a diet that conflicts with your daily routine. Although intermittent fasting (IF) has a number of health benefits, it is not for everyone.

You may find it difficult to adhere to an intermittent fasting schedule if you are the type of person who basically consumes small amounts of food or snacks throughout the day. According to Dana White, RD, losing weight is not recommended for individuals with a history of easily eating disorders, diabetes, or who are pregnant or breastfeeding. This is true regardless of whether dieting is encouraged. In addition, if your schedule is unpredictable or if you exercise at different times of the day, you should likely reconsider the possibility of beginning IF.

If you have a history of nighttime binge easily eating or are looking to easily increase your level of self-discipline, intermittent fasting may help you avoid mindless easily eating during the day. If you have previously attempted to create a calorie deficit without success, this may also be a viable option for you.

According to White, the 16:8 method is the most prevalent (there is more information about this method below). On the other hand, there are an abundance of alternative options. Here are the six most common IF strategies for weight loss, as well as what the most recent research says about the potential same benefits or drawbacks of each of these approaches individually. In all seriousness, the diet that is most likely to be successful for you is the one that you can adhere to, so the IF plan that appears to be the easiest to follow is your best option.

The 16:8 method of intermittent fasting involves abstaining from food for a total of 16 hours per day and restricting easily eating to eight hours. This schedule requires the majority of individuals to abstain from easily eating after dinner and in the morning. You might basically consume food between noon and eight o'clock at night.

If you are the type of person who prefers to complete your workouts first thing in the morning, White suggests selecting an alternative program that is more accommodating (see the 14:10 diet). If, on the other hand, you prefer to schedule your workouts for the late afternoon or after 5:00 p.m., you will still have time to easy eat a meal to refuel after your workout.

How does the 16:8 technique for weight loss fare in terms of effectiveness? The (extremely limited) research indicates that success is possible. In a study published in the journal Nutrition and Healthy Aging, 23 obese male and female participants followed the 16:8 diet for a duration of 12 weeks. Those who followed the 16:8 diet basically consumed 350 fewer calories per day than a control group that ate normally and not according to a predetermined schedule. In addition, they experienced modest weight loss (approximately three percent of their body weight on average) and a decrease in blood pressure. However, it is important to remember that this was a small study, and there isn't much research on the 16:8 diet in particular, so it is difficult to say that adhering to the 16:8 diet is a foolproof way to lose weight.

The 5:2 Diet Plan

The 5:2 diet requires that you easy eat normally for five days of the week and then basically consume 20 percent of your typical daily caloric intake for the remaining two days of the week. On days of fasting, women are restricted to approximately 500 calories, while men are permitted approximately 600. If you choose to implement this strategy, you must basically consume a healthy meal the day prior to your fast in order to avoid binge easily eating when it is finally time to easy eat again.

As long as your body is functioning normally, you continue to burn calories even when you are at rest. During sleep, the body utilizes glycogen stored in the liver to maintain steady blood sugar levels. This indicates that your body is accustomed to the metabolic processes that occur during fasting.

Your body is designed to compensate for the lack of energy provided by meals. The purpose of practices such as fasting is to lengthen the period of time during which your body is forced to rely solely on its reserve energy reserves as opposed to consuming external sources of energy.

This intermittent fasting strategy results in the same amount of weight and fat loss for its participants as conventional dieting methods.

Chapter 9: The Intermittent Fasting Mimicking Diet

As the name suggests, this diet mimics intermittent fasting but it is less strict compared to IF. With this diet, you will basically consume small portions of food during the fasting period. The food eaten during the fasting period is usually 40% of the calories you normally basically consume.

The average duration of this mimicking diet is five days. Participants in the mimicking diet claim that it provides the majority of the same benefits of intermittent fasting without the stress of total abstinence from food.

People who are not accustomed to abstaining from food for longer than 12 hours may find intermittent fasting to be extremely difficult. The mimicking diet provides a less strict alternative.

Since this diet allows you to restrict your calorie intake for no more than 5 days, you don't need to worry about losing out on essential nutrients.

People on the diet that mimics intermittent fasting are encouraged to repeasy eat it twice or four times per year. If they really want to do this frequently, they should limit themselves to once per month.

How Does It Function?

This diet is strictly vegetarian, gluten-free, and lactose-free. You must basically consume between 700 and 1200 calories per day for the next five days. It is best to start with a higher calorie count (1200 calories) at the beginning of the fast and gradually reduce it as your body gets used to it.

During this period, your body will start to burn fat as fuel resulting in weight loss.

Combining Intermittent Fasting and Exercise Mimicking diet and Intermittent Fasting?

Since you are expected to basically consume a small number of calories regardless, combining these two is even simpler. Simply basically consume these meals when you break your fast, and refrain from easily eating between meals.

You will need to schedule your meals around your fasting schedule. For instance, if you are using the 16:8 intermittent fasting schedule, restrict your meals to the 8-hour easily eating window.

You should be aware, however, that the diet mimicking is a short-term diet. Going beyond the 5-day limit is neither beneficial nor safe. After five days, your body will adapt to this easily eating schedule and enter a state of starvation.

It will reduce metabolic rate and store glucose for later use. Therefore, it will not burn as much fat. Most people use the Intermittent fasting mimicking diet as an introduction to intermittent fasting.

SUGAR WITHDRAWAL STAGE Although the list of common withdrawal symptoms may be intimidating, keep in mind that they are temporary and typically only last a few days for most people. Here are the challenges you will face if you decide to eliminate sugar from your diet:

1. feeling inspired

When you decide to eliminate sugar from your diet, you will likely feel highly motivated and prepared to reap the same benefits of a healthier diet and way of life. You'll need this motivation to just get you through the hunger, headache, and exhaustion that lie ahead.

2. Cravings Start to Kisk Sugar withdrawal is characterized by cravings as one of its earliest symptoms. Many people, for example, establish a routine with their diet, and many find themselves glancing at the vending machine when hunger strikes in the middle of the morning.

During this season, it is best to keep healthy snacks on hand to make it easier to resist the temptation to indulge in your favorite sweets.

3. Symptoms You may begin to experience some of the previously mentioned sugar withdrawal symptoms soon after your cravings peak. Headache, hunger, chills, and even sugar withdrawal diarrhea can make it more difficult than ever to tau motivate oneself.

Remember why you decided to easy eat healthier, and use that to keep you motivated and determined to continue on the path to better health.

You begin to feel better.

As soon as your symptoms begin to clear up, you will likely feel better than ever. As a result of giving up added sugar, numerous individuals have reported improvements in skin health, diminished brain fog, and increased energy.

In addition, by adhering to a healthy diet and consuming more nutrient-dense foods, you will reduce your risk of developing cardiovascular disease and improve your overall health.

Chapter 10: What's the Difference Between Becoming Fitter and Losing Fat?

When you observe the numbers on your scale decrease, you may feel energized. However, the scale does not indicate that you have lost fat or weight overall. You may believe that the purpose of your fitness program is to really become physically fit, but what you really need is to reduce your muscle-to-fat ratio. The explanation is simple: when you just get in shape, you can lose a combination of muscle, liquids, fat, and organ size.

To improve your health and add muscle so that your body feels and appears toned, losing muscle and fluids is probably not your goal. In the end, you'll need to zero in on fat loss, so losing more than two pounds per week could be detrimental to your goals.

According to research and Specialist Joel Seedman, when you lose up to five pounds per week, you will also lose water weight and muscle in addition to fat. Muscle and water loss can be dangerous because it puts you at risk for dehydration, nutrient deficiencies, deteriorating health and mental performance, and weight regain. To combat this, incorporate strength training into your daily gym routine. Aerobic exercise can aid in fat loss, but resistance training is essential for maintaining muscle mass. Similarly, the greater your mass, the greater your metabolic rate. Basic strength-training exercises, such as squats, sprints, and push-ups, can build muscle and enhance muscle-versus-fat synthesis.

Chapter 11: What Advantages Does Intermittent Fasting Offer?

Several studies indicate that intermittent fasting may aid in weight loss, memory and mental performance improvement, cardiovascular health, type 2 diabetes management, and cancer treatment effectiveness.

Even though the majority of this research is based on animal studies, recent advances in human research have shown promising results, particularly in terms of the potential to aid in weight loss and ameliorate certain nutrition-related chronic diseases such as diabetes and heart disease.

Although the long-term effects of intermittent fasting have not yet been thoroughly investigated, recent research has revealed a number of promising short-term benefits, which we have outlined below. Although the potential same benefits of fasting are intriguing, there is insufficient evidence to conclude that it is superior to healthy easily eating for weight loss or health improvement.

It is common knowledge that easily eating in moderation or excess has a much greater impact on weight loss than easily eating frequently or at specific times. However, intermittent fasting may allow you to maintain a caloric deficit that leads to weight loss.

However, intermittent fasting alone does not necessarily indicate a calorie deficit. Some individuals have difficulty remaining within a healthy calorie range, even when they limit the duration of their meals. Utilize this calculator to determine a safe caloric range for your diet and lifestyle.

It has been demonstrated that calorie restriction can reduce body weight and visceral fat, but it can be difficult to maintain a healthy caloric deficit over long periods of time. Intermittent fasting is regarded as an effective weight loss strategy in light of recent human studies demonstrating significant decreases in body weight and visceral fat.

Intermittent fasting is a difficult intervention to investigate over the long term due to the difficulty of encouraging individuals to reduce their food intake while fasting and the potential influence of variables such as protein intake, length of fasting, and food quality on results. It is unknown if yo-yo dieting or weight gain will occur after fasting is terminated; therefore, additional research is required to evaluate any long-term weight loss same benefits of intermittent fasting.

Intermittent fasting may result in greater weight loss than calorie restriction alone. Fasting-induced physiological changes, such as lower levels of the hormones leptin and insulin, may result in greater weight loss than calorie restriction alone.

Ultimately, maintaining a healthy weight requires more than calorie restriction techniques such as intermittent fasting. Our ability to lose and maintain weight depends on a variety of factors, such as our lifestyle, stress levels, and sleep patterns, among others.

Intermittent fasting may aid in weight loss, which may also affect other fasting benefits.

By decreasing leptin concentrations — a hormone produced by fat cells that regulates hunger — and increasing adiponectin, a hormone involved in glucose and lipid metabolism, intermittent fasting and weight loss may help reduce fasting blood glucose and improve insulin sensitivity.

People who intermittently fasted in clinical trials where fasting was used as a weight-loss intervention and method of maintaining a healthy weight had lower blood glucose levels, which is a key goal in the prevention and treatment of diabetes.

Although evidence indicates that intermittent fasting has a generally positive impact on blood sugar levels, these potential same benefits could be impacted more by calorie restriction-induced reductions in body weight and body fat percentage.

Intermittent fasting may help those with and without diabetes lose weight and improve their glycemic control and insulin sensitivity.

Following intermittent fasting, if you basically consume a nutritious diet when you are not fasting, your cholesterol may also decrease. In healthy and obese individuals, intermittent fasting has been associated with improved lipid profiles, including decreased total cholesterol, LDL (low-density lipoprotein), and triglyceride levels.

As the majority of studies examining its effects have been conducted on Ramadan fasters, intermittent fasting may be a useful dietary strategy for reducing cholesterol. However, additional research is necessary to fully comprehend the distinctions between the short-term and long-term metabolic changes caused by fasting.

Consider adopting healthy lifestyle habits, such as regular exercise and a diet rich in high-fiber, low-saturated-fat foods, if high cholesterol is a concern.

Chapter 12: How To Effectively Commence Intermittent Fasting

Although fasting is generally safe for most healthy, well-nourished individuals, it may not be appropriate for those with medical conditions. The purpose of the following guidelines is to make fasting as simple and effective as possible for individuals whose doctors deem them eligible to do so safely.

1. Establish Individual Objectives

A person who begins intermittent fasting typically has a specific goal in mind. It could be to lose weight, improve overall health, or enhance metabolic health. The final objective of a person will help them select the optimal fasting method and determine how many calories and nutrients they need to basically consume.

2. Select the method

While fasting for health reasons, a person may explore numerous possible approaches. They should adopt a strategy that satisfies their preferences and that they believe they can successfully implement.

Before attempting a new fasting strategy, a person should typically adhere to one method for a minimum of one month to determine if it is effective. Before beginning a fasting program, anyone with a medical condition should consult a medical professional. For some individuals, fasting is an unsafe option.

A person should keep in mind that they do not need to basically consume a specific amount or type of food or completely avoid certain foods when selecting a strategy. Following an intermittent fasting strategy, a person may basically consume whatever they wish.

To achieve health and weight management goals, it is advisable to basically consume a balanced, high-protein, high-fiber, and vegetable-rich diet at all mealtimes.

Consuming only meals devoid of beneficial nutrients during mealtimes may hinder health improvement. During fasting, it is also vitally important to basically consume copious amounts of water or other non-caloric liquids.

3. Figure out calorie needs

Intermittent fasting has no inherent dietary restrictions, but this does not imply that calories do not matter.

Those who are working with a physician or nutritionist to maintain a healthy weight must create a calorie deficit by consuming fewer calories than they burn. People who wish to gain weight must basically consume more calories than they burn.

Numerous tools are available to assist individuals in calculating their calorie needs and determining how many calories they should basically consume daily in order to gain, lose, or maintain weight.

A person may also seek advice from a healthcare professional or dietician regarding the number of calories they need. A professional may assist a person in identifying the optimal foods for weight loss and developing an overall health strategy.

4. Develop a diet plan

A person interested in losing or gaining weight may find it beneficial to plan their daily or weekly dietary intake.

Meal preparation need not be extremely restrictive. It evaluates caloric intake and incorporates sufficient nutrients into the diet. For instance, the Centers for Disease Control and Prevention (CDC) endorses the MyPlatePlan, which focuses on providing daily dietary category goals.

Meal planning has numerous benefits, such as helping a person adhere to their calorie restriction and ensuring they have the necessary ingredients for recipes, quick dinners, and snacks. Meal planning could potentially save money if it helps individuals waste less food.

5. Keep track of calorie intake

Not all calories are created equal. Despite the fact that these fasting methods do not limit the number of calories a person basically consumes during mealtimes, it is essential to evaluate the nutritional value of the food.

In general, a person should strive to basically consume nutrient-dense or high-nutrient-to-calorie ratio meals. They may not have to completely abstain from less nutritious meals, but they should still practice moderation and focus on more nutritious foods to obtain the greatest benefits.

Chapter 13: Potential Danger Factors Associated With Intermittent Fasting

Some individuals may be more prone to binge easily eating when not fasting if they experience hunger during their fasting period. In addition, even if you consistently fast for 12 to 16 hours per day, consuming more calories than your body uses will result in a gradual easily increase in body fat.

In other words, you run the risk of gaining weight if you struggle to control your hunger and end up binging during non-fasting periods. Establish a meal-preparation routine or schedule your meals to ensure that you are fueling your body during non-fasting periods, as going rogue during these times can compromise your health goals.

Intermittent fasting does not replace healthy easily eating or calorie restriction; you can still gain weight if you basically consume more calories than your body uses while fasting.

When you fast for an extended period of time, your blood sugar levels drop, which can result in headaches, nausea, lightheadedness, and/or dizziness.

If you have a medical condition, consult your doctor to determine if intermittent fasting is safe for you to try. Those with type 1 diabetes who take diabetic medications or who have the disease themselves may be more susceptible to adverse side effects or have difficulty controlling their blood sugar.

Choose a day of the week or time when you won't need to be particularly active or attentive when beginning a fasting regimen, as your body will need time to acclimate.

3. Restrictive Easily eating Can Influence Easily eating Disorders

Any diet that encourages skipping meals or restricting food intake can result in negative associations with food. Especially when restricting or skipping meals negatively impacts weight loss results.

This is a poor mindset to enter fasting with, as it may lead some individuals to go too far, develop disordered easily eating patterns, or fall victim to yo-yo dieting.

Insufficient daily caloric intake may also result in vitamin deficiencies, a weakened immune system, and other health issues.

Be truthful with yourself prior to attempting any type of fasting practice, as a mindful or intuitive easily eating approach may be a better option. Additionally, you should consult your practitioner first.

Regardless of your motivation for attempting an intermittent fast, you must combine basic nutrition principles such as calorie restriction and a balanced diet to ensure your success.

Your hopes of reaping the health same benefits of intermittent fasting may be dashed if you stray from your diet during non-fasting periods.

After consuming a large amount of food in one sitting during their easily eating windows, some individuals may experience intestinal pain. This may include digestive symptoms such as gas, cramps, indigestion, and bloating. However, because each individual's body is unique, experiencing digestive symptoms as a result of intermittent fasting is highly individualized. Nonetheless, it is essential to remember this if intermittent fasting significantly alters your easily eating pattern or the amount of food you basically consume at once.

Due to their sensitivity and propensity for inflammation, individuals with irritable bowel syndrome may not be suitable candidates for intermittent fasting. These individuals are consequently more susceptible to cramping, bloating, and abdominal pain.

If intermittent fasting and exercise cause an individual to feel uncomfortably hungry, they may basically consume more food than usual when their easily eating window finally opens. It actually depends on your individual hunger and fullness cues, despite the fact that intermittent fasting can work without increasing hunger for some individuals.

If you just get hungry later in the day and find that three larger meals leave you feeling more satisfied, intermittent fasting may be a better option for you. However, if you prefer to basically consume smaller, more frequent meals throughout the day and experience hunger in the morning and evening, intermittent fasting may easily increase your hunger during the fasting windows.

This drawback of intermittent fasting is most likely to affect leaner individuals (those with less weight to lose) and those with active lifestyles. As mentioned in the previous paragraph, hormonal imbalances can result in irregular menstrual cycles for women, lower testosterone levels in men, as well as more instances of insomnia and higher reported levels of stress across the board, regardless of gender. People who are obese and practice intermittent fasting are more likely to gain same benefits and lose a greater percentage of body fat during the fast.

Realistically, intermittent fasting is not always compatible with daily responsibilities and can be difficult to maintain. If you have a family, it can be agonizing to prepare meals for others during your fasting window.

In addition, it is not always possible to decline breakfast or dinner meetings that conflict with your self-imposed easily eating window.

Traveling for business or pleasure can also disrupt your easily eating schedule

by disrupting your circadian rhythms
and leaving you famished at inopportune
times.

Chapter 14: Achieving Hormonal Harmony

Hormones have a substantial effect on your mental, physical, and emotional health. For example, they play a significant role in regulating your mood, appetite, and weight.

Typically, your body produces the precise amount of each hormone required for various processes to maintain health. However, sedentary lifestyles and Western easily eating habits may have an impact on your hormonal environment. In addition, as people age, their levels of various hormones decline, although some people experience a more pronounced decline than others.

However, a healthy diet and other health-promoting lifestyle choices could help you feel and perform at your best by enhancing your hormonal balance. However, a nutritious diet and other healthy lifestyle choices may improve your hormonal health and allow you to perform at your peak.

Here are a few natural hormone balance remedies.

Ensure that you basically consume sufficient protein at each meal. These hormones are produced by your endocrine glands using amino acids. Numerous physiological processes, including growth, energy metabolism, appetite, stress, and reproduction, are regulated by peptide hormones. Protein consumption, for instance, affects the hormones that regulate appetite and food intake, thereby providing the brain with information about energy level.

Studies show that easily eating protein reduces the hunger hormone ghrelin and increases the release of hormones that make you feel full. Therefore, experts recommend consuming at least 20-30 grams of protein per meal. This can be accomplished by easily eating high-protein foods at each meal, such as eggs, chicken breast, lentils, and seafood.

2. Take frequent exercise. Physical activity has a significant influence on hormonal health. By increasing the sensitivity of your hormone receptors, exercise promotes the passage of nutrients and hormone signals, while also increasing blood flow to your muscles. Significant benefit is exercise's ability to easily increase insulin sensitivity and decrease insulin levels. Insulin enables cells to absorb glucose

from the bloodstream and use it as fuel. Nonetheless, if you develop a disease known as insulin resistance, your cells may not respond to insulin.

This condition is a risk factor for cardiovascular disease, diabetes, and obesity. Regular exercise may reduce insulin resistance regardless of body weight, although some studies are still debating whether the effects result from exercise itself or from weight loss or fat mass reduction. Several physical activities, including high-intensity interval training, weight training, and cardio, have been reported to help prevent insulin resistance.

Physical activity may easily increase the levels of hormones that maintain muscle mass, such as testosterone, which decline with age. Those unable to engage in strenuous exercise can easily increase these hormone levels by simply walking, which may improve their quality of life and strength.

Maintain a healthy weight gain:

Is directly associated with hormonal abnormalities that may cause complications in insulin sensitivity and fecundity.

Obesity is inextricably linked to the progression of insulin resistance, whereas weight loss is associated with improvements in insulin deterrent and a lower risk of diabetes.

Obesity ailment Weight is also associated with hypogonadism, which is a decrease or absence of hormone secretion from the gonads or ovaries.

In fact, this condition is one of the most significant hormonal complexities of male heaviness. This suggests that obesity is strongly associated with lower levels of the sperm-stimulating hormone testosterone in men and contributes to a lack of ovulation in women, both of which are typical causes of futility.

4. Take care of your stomach health

Your stomach contains more than 100 trillion beneficial microorganisms that produce numerous metabolites that may affect your chemical health in both positive and negative ways.

Your stomach microbiome controls chemicals by regulating insulin obstruction and feelings of completeness.

When your stomach microbiome ferments fiber, for instance, it produces short-chain unsaturated fatty acids (SCFAs) such as acetic acid derivation, propionate, and butyrate. Both acetic acid derivation and butyrate help the board gain weight by increasing calorie consumption and thereby aid in preventing insulin obstruction.

Curiously, research demonstrates that obesity may alter the stomach microbiome to advance insulin obstruction and inflammation.

In addition, lipopolysaccharides (LPS), which are components of specific microorganisms in your stomach microbiome, may easily increase your risk of insulin resistance. Individuals who are overweight appear to have higher LPS levels in the bloodstream.

5. Cut back on your sugar intake

Increasing chemical capacity and preventing weight gain, diabetes, and other diseases may be facilitated by limiting added sugar consumption.

The simple sugar fructose is present in numerous sugars, with up to 43% of honey, 50% of refined table sugar, 55%

of high fructose corn syrup, and 90% of agave containing fructose.

Also, sugar-enhanced beverages are the primary source of added sugars in the Western diet, and fructose is typically used commercially in sodas, fruit juice, and alcoholic and caffeinated beverages.

Since 1980, fructose consumption has increased dramatically in the United States, and research consistently demonstrates that easily eating added sugar increases insulin resistance — regardless of calorie intake or weight gain.

Long-term fructose consumption has been linked to alterations in the microbiome of the stomach, which may cause other hormonal imbalances.

Additionally, fructose may not stimulate the production of the endogenous chemical leptin, resulting in decreased calorie consumption and increased weight gain. Consequently, reducing your consumption of sugary beverages and other sources of added sugar can promote chemical health.

6. Attempt pressure decrease procedures

Stress harms your body's chemicals in multiple ways.

Cortisol is known as the pressure chemical because it assists the body in adapting to prolonged stress.

Your body's response to stress triggers an abundance of events that induce cortisol production. When the stressor is no longer present, the reaction ends. However, persistent stress debilitates the input mechanisms that restore your hormonal systems to normal.

Constant pressure causes cortisol levels to remain elevated, which stimulates cravings and increases your intake of sweet and high-fat foods. Thus, this may result in excessive calorie consumption and weight gain.

Similarly, elevated cortisol levels stimulate gluconeogenesis, the production of glucose from non-starch sources, which may result in insulin resistance.

In fact, research demonstrates that you can reduce your cortisol levels by engaging in stress-reduction activities such as meditation, yoga, and listening to soothing music.

Try to devote at least 10 to 15 minutes per day to these exercises, regardless of whether you believe you have the time or energy to do so.

7. Obtain regular, superior rest

Regardless of the quality of your diet or the regularity of your exercise routine, getting sufficient rest is essential for optimal health.

A large number of hormones, including insulin, cortisol, leptin, ghrelin, and HGH, are linked to unlucky sleep, including insulin, cortisol, leptin, ghrelin, and HGH.

In contrast, poor rest is associated with a 24-hour easily increase in cortisol levels, which can result in insulin obstruction. In fact, a small study of 14 healthy adults found that five nights of sleep restriction decreased insulin sensitivity by 25%. In addition, consistent evidence indicates that lack of sleep increases ghrelin and decreases leptin levels. In a survey of 21 tests on 2,250 individuals, those assigned to a short rest group had higher ghrelin levels than those who received the recommended amount of rest.

In addition, your mind requires continuous rest to pass through all five phases of each rest cycle. This is especially important for the release of development chemicals, which occurs primarily in the evening during deep sleep. To maintain optimal hormonal balance, just get seven hours of quality sleep every night.

Chapter 15: Utilizing Intermittent Fasting To Accelerate Anti-Aging

calorie restriction improves energy production and reduces the risk of chronic diseases such as cancer, diabetes, and heart disease.

Calorie restriction reduces cellular deterioration and promotes the maintenance of healthy DNA. Chronic disease is caused by damaged and inflamed cells, whereas aging is caused by DNA degradation; therefore, these are two essential components in the fight against aging.

Although it has been demonstrated that calorie restriction has anti-aging benefits, the majority of people cannot adhere to a diet that requires a 30–40% reduction in daily caloric intake for an extended period of time.

Rapidly, intermittent fasting as an alternative to calorie restriction gained popularity. It provides the same life extension same benefits without imposing dietary restrictions.

Results of aging

Fasting increases the body's ability to digest food and burn calories by accelerating the metabolism. As a result, the aging process is slowed. Additionally, it accelerates DNA repair and prevents the aging-related DNA degradation.

Fasting also increases antioxidants, which can help protect the body's cells from free radicals, which can be harmful to cells. Additionally, fasting can reduce the chronic inflammation associated with aging. Intermittent fasting extends and improves the quality of human life. Regardless of the duration or frequency of the fast, the body undergoes positive changes during fasting. Intermittent fasting induces the following changes, all of which help people live longer and healthier lives:

In the process of cell repair, cells easily increase the removal of potentially harmful wastes.
The expression of genes: Genes that prolong life and prevent disease vary.

Hormonal alterations: Lower insulin levels prevent diabetes and may easily increase life expectancy.
Infrequently does fasting decrease inflammation.
Reduces oxidative stress: prevents cell degeneration caused by unstable chemicals known as free radicals.
In addition, losing weight and abdominal fat through intermittent fasting improves your health and protects you from chronic diseases that can shorten your life span.

Chapter 16: What Is Allowed During Intermittent Fasting, And What Makes Fasting Possible?

Intermittent fasting is the practice of alternating between periods of easily eating and fasting. But during a fast, is nothing permissible to basically consume? How about a cup of tea or coffee in the morning? Specifically, what ends a fast?

What is permitted during a fast is determined by the intermittent fasting (IF) type chosen and the goals being pursued.

In general, during time-restricted intermittent fasting, you basically consume nothing but calorie-dense liquids such as water, unsweetened coffee, and tea without milk. When you are not fasting, it is essential to maintain a healthy, well-balanced diet. Many individuals adhere to IF in an effort to improve their health. According to some studies, a prolonged fast may be advantageous because it forces the body to switch from burning sugar to burning fat for energy.

Is it truly necessary to abstain from easily eating and drinking during all meals? Depending on your chosen strategy. On fasting days of the 5:2 diet with alternate-day fasting, you basically consume fewer calories. During the fasting period of time-restricted eating, you typically abstain from all foods and liquids. Your body converts the food you basically consume into sugar or glucose for energy. When food and, consequently, glucose are unavailable for an extended period of time, the body breaks down fat to produce ketones, an alternative energy source. Alternating between easily eating and fasting or utilizing glucose and ketones for energy may be advantageous.

Technically, breaking a fast involves consuming calories. This indicates that water and unsweetened black coffee or tea are commonly accepted as acceptable beverages.

However, some of the potential same benefits of fasting may be a result of avoiding certain metabolic processes, such as a rise in blood sugar levels. What does this imply for the milk in your morning coffee?

Even though everyone reacts differently to food, for the vast majority of individuals, the amount of milk in tea or coffee is insufficient to raise blood sugar levels. If you are fasting, you should avoid artificial sweeteners because they may cause your blood sugar to rise or fall.

Technically, there are no restrictions on the types of meals that may be basically consumed outside of fasting. To preserve gut health, regulate lipid and blood sugar responses, and prevent dietary inflammation, food quality is indispensable.

Easily eating a balanced, nutritious diet will improve your overall health. If you easy eat a variety of vegetables, the good bacteria in your gut will be nourished and your body will receive the necessary nutrients. If you basically consume protein and fiber from trustworthy sources, you may feel fuller for longer. Include as many whole grains, fresh fruits and vegetables, fish, poultry, lentils, nuts, and seeds as possible, along with legumes such as peas and lentils. Your intermittent fasting goals may also influence what you choose to basically consume. as an instance;

According to Martin, "frequently, people begin a new easily eating regimen, such as a fasting diet, at the same time they begin a new exercise program or easily increase the intensity of their current exercise program." Even if you exercise very intensely, it is possible that you will basically consume more calories during your easily eating windows than you will burn off.

How to remedy the situation: On days when you are performing full-day fasts, such as when following the 5:2 method, you should perform relatively light exercise. "Generally, you should aim to make your exercise regimen challenging, while also ensuring that it is manageable and enjoyable. If you have an insatiable appetite on exercise days, it may indicate that you are exceeding your limits "says Martin.

If you do not drink enough water during your fast, you run the risk of becoming dehydrated; in addition, you will not receive the appetite-suppressing same benefits of water because you will not be drinking enough water.

Drink a lot of water to solve the issue! Additionally, you have the option to flavor your water. During an intermittent fast, the following beverages are permitted: hot tea, black coffee, seltzer water, iced tea, and either tea or coffee sweetened with Stevia.

According to Smith, "Following an intermittent fasting plan can be challenging for some dieters because they aren't used to going for long periods of time without eating." Therefore, if you continue to deviate from your diet plan from week to week or look for shortcuts, you should expect that your efforts will not result in the weight loss you had hoped for. Consequently, you may wish to reconsider whether or not intermittent fasting is suitable for your lifestyle.

According to Smith, the solution is to select an intermittent fasting plan that is compatible with your lifestyle and can be adhered to for extended periods.

According to Smith, "planning ahead is essential for maintaining any type of healthy intervention," and this is true for any type of healthy intervention.

The following is the answer: "Make an effort to plan at least one day in advance for all of your meals and snacks." Smith recommends having a plan for what you will prepare, such as bringing your own meals and snacks or reviewing restaurant menus in advance to decide what to order.

Practice and perseverance are required for IF. According to Martin, "the majority of people who experiment with intermittent fasting will break a fast ahead of schedule at some point," regardless of the strategy they employ. "If you are serious about continuing intermittent fasting, it is important not to feel guilty, ashamed, or angry at yourself for doing so, and to return as soon as possible to a regularly scheduled program." "If you are serious about continuing IF, it is important to not feel guilty, ashamed, or mad at yourself for doing so."

The best solution to this issue is to extend yourself some grace and move on with your life.

" It's important to remember that intermittent fasting requires some trial and error; it's inevitable that your IF schedule won't always go as planned, so it's important to be flexible, " says Martin.

Chapter 17: Aspects Of Intermittent Fasting

The fact that IF can be implemented in so many different ways is a very positive development. If you are interested in pursuing this course of action, you can determine the approach that is most compatible with your lifestyle, which will significantly easily increase your chances of success. Here are seven:

1. Abstain for twelve hours per day

Numerous variations of the intermittent fasting lifestyle may be successful.

The instructions for following this diet are straightforward. Every day, an individual must choose and adhere to a 12-hour fasting window.

According to the findings of certain researchers, fasting for 10 to 16 hours may allow the body to convert its fat stores into energy, resulting in the release of ketones into the bloodstream. This should encourage individuals to lose weight.

It is possible that intermittent fasting could be beneficial for those who are just getting started. This is because the time spent fasting is very brief, the majority of the time spent fasting occurs while the individual is asleep, and they can basically consume the same amount of calories daily.

If you really want to complete the 12-hour fast as efficiently as possible, you should include your sleep time in the fasting window.

For instance, a person may choose to abstain from food and drink between the hours of 7 p.m. and 7 a.m. They would have to finish dinner by 7 p.m., but breakfast would not be available until 7 a.m. However, they would spend the majority of their time between meals and sleep sleeping.

16-hour fasting

The 16:8 technique, also known as the Leangains diet, consists of fasting for 16 hours per day and allowing yourself an 8-hour easily eating window.

Men are required to fast for 16 hours per day on the 16:8 diet, while women fast for 14 hours. A person who has previously tried the 12-hour fast but did not experience any same benefits may find that intermittent fasting is more beneficial.

On this type of fast, participants typically finish their evening meal by 8:00 p.m., then skip breakfast the following day, delaying their next meal until 12:00 p.m.

Even though they basically consumed the same total number of calories as mice that were permitted to easy eat whenever they pleased, mice that were easily given an eight-hour feeding window were protected from obesity, inflammation, diabetes, and liver disease. This was the conclusion of a study conducted with mice.

2. fasting twice per week

People adhering to the 5:2 diet basically consume the same amount of nutritious food as usual for five days, but reduce their caloric intake for the final two days.

In general, men basically consume 600 calories during a two-day fast, whereas women basically consume only 500 calories.

Typically, people distribute their fasting days across the seven days of the week. They may, for example, abstain from food on Mondays and Thursdays but basically consume normally on the other days of the week. In between cycles of the fasting regimen, a minimum of one day of rest is required.

The 5:2 diet, also known as the Fast diet, has received a limited amount of academic attention. In a study involving 107 overweight or obese women, both intermittent calorie restriction twice weekly and continuous calorie restriction were found to lead to the same amount of weight loss.

As a result of following this diet, insulin levels were found to be lower, and insulin sensitivity was reported to have increased.

Twenty-three obese women were examined to determine the effects of this particular type of fasting by researchers. Over the course of a single menstrual cycle, the ladies lost 4.8% of their total body weight and 8.0% of their total body fat. After five days of returning to a normal easily eating pattern, however, these measurements returned to normal for the majority of the women.

Alternating day of fasting

The plan of fasting every other day, also known as the alternate-day fasting plan, can be implemented in a variety of ways.

On the fasting days of alternate day fasting, some individuals abstain entirely from solid foods, while others basically consume up to 500 calories. On feeding days, individuals frequently choose to easy eat whatever they want, whenever they want.

According to research, alternating day fasting is effective for promoting weight loss and preserving heart health in both healthy and overweight individuals. Over the course of a year, the researchers discovered that each of the 32 subjects lost an average of 5.2

kilograms (kg), or roughly 11 pounds (lb).

Alternate-day fasting is a relatively strenuous form of intermittent fasting, and those who are new to fasting or who have certain medical conditions may wish to avoid it. It could be difficult to maintain this type of fasting over an extended period of time.

5. A 24-hour weekly fast

On a 24-hour diet, it is permissible to basically consume devoid-of-calorie teas and other beverages.

The Eat-Stop-Easy eat diet consists of abstaining from food consumption for a period of twenty-four hours once per week. On consecutive days, a significant number of individuals skip either breakfast or lunch.

During the time they are supposed to be fasting, adherents of this diet plan are permitted to basically consume calorie-free beverages such as water, tea, and others.

On days when fasting is not required, individuals should resume their normal easily eating habits. Consuming meals in this manner reduces an individual's overall caloric intake without restricting the types of foods they basically consume.

A twenty-four hour fast may be difficult and may cause symptoms such as fatigue, headaches, and irritation. As the body adjusts to the new easily eating pattern, many individuals discover that these symptoms diminish over time.

Prior to embarking on a 24-hour fast, it may be advantageous for individuals to try fasting for 12 or 16 hours.

6. Meal skipping

This variable approach to intermittent fasting could prove beneficial for beginners. This strategy requires occasional meal skipping.

People have the option of skipping meals based on how hungry they are or the amount of time they have. However, it is necessary to basically consume healthy foods at every meal.

People have the best chance of successfully skipping meals if they are attentive to and responsive to the hunger cues their bodies send. Followers of this method of intermittent fasting will, for the most part, easy eat only when they are hungry and skip meals when they are not hungry.

Some individuals may find this method of fasting easier on their bodies than others.

The Warrior Diet 7. (Warrior Diet)

The Warrior Diet is a form of intermittent fasting that is regarded as one of the strictest on the spectrum.

The Warrior Diet consists of easily eating very little during a 20-hour fasting window, typically just a few servings of raw fruits and vegetables, and then consuming a massive meal at night. The purpose of this is to maximize fat loss. Typically, the window of opportunity to basically consume food is no longer than four hours.

Those who have already experimented with other forms of intermittent fasting may derive the most benefit from this method.

Followers of the Warrior Diet assert that humans are naturally nocturnal eaters and that consuming food at night allows the body to obtain the nutrients it needs in a manner that is in sync with its circadian rhythms.

During the four-hour easily eating period, individuals should basically consume a substantial amount of vegetables, proteins, and fats that are healthy for their bodies. In addition, carbohydrates must be present.

Even though it is possible to basically consume some foods during the fasting period, it can be challenging to adhere to the stringent basically requirements regarding when and what types of foods can be basically consumed. In addition, some individuals have difficulty falling asleep after consuming such a substantial dinner so close to bedtime.

People who adhere to this diet run the risk of not consuming enough of certain nutrients, such as fiber. In addition to increasing the risk of developing cancer, this can have negative effects on the health of the digestive system and the immune system.

Chapter 18: It Is All About The Timing

There are numerous possible schedules for intermittent fasting. When following a weekly intermittent fasting program, you limit your consumption to three days per week. Another type of fasting is time-restricted feeding, which is exactly what it sounds like: you restrict your daily food intake to a certain number of hours and fast for the remainder. According to research, both strategies can aid in weight loss, easily increase metabolic efficiency, and reduce the risk of diabetes and obesity. (Women who are pregnant or breastfeeding or who have a history of easily eating disorders should avoid fasting.)

It has been shown that intermittent fasting alters the microbiome's composition. Your gut flora is highly sensitive to food availability and absence. When food is removed from the microbiome, the composition of the microbiome alters. According to studies, the circadian rhythm of the microbiome cycles continuously across populations. It is hypothesized that a certain type of bacteria thrives in humans when they are sleeping and not eating. When you begin to eat, other plants may sprout and take over. The cycle repeats every twenty-four hours, though it can be disrupted by irregular easily eating or a poor diet.

Time-restricted meals can reinforce and aid in the restoration of these naturally occurring fluctuations. Two of the most popular intermittent fasting patterns are 16:8, in which you fast for 16 hours and easy eat for the remaining 8, and 5:2, in which you easy eat normally for five days of the week and then severely restrict your caloric intake for two consecutive days.

If you really want to observe changes at the cellular or microbial level, you must lengthen the fasting duration. However, fasting days are not required to be calorie-free. On fasting days, the majority of diet plans prescribe a 70–75 percent reduction in caloric intake; however, even a 60 percent reduction can be effective.

During feeding periods, you should not restrict your caloric intake; the majority of your intestinal microbes require food to thrive. When your body enters starvation mode, such as when you fast for too long, the diversity of bacteria in your gut decreases. For this reason, she recommends that fasting be "really intermittent" and that you never fast for more than two days consecutively.

Fasting on a 24-hour cycle permits you to synchronize your fasting with your natural sleep/wake cycles. This is significant easily given that circadian rhythms regulate nutrient digestion. The morning and midday hours are when insulin sensitivity is at its peak. Nevertheless, hormones such as melatonin inhibit insulin action in the evening and at night. If you basically consume a snack late at night, the insulin you secrete to help metabolize it will not function.

Because insulin is responsible for transporting sugar from the blood into the cells, your blood sugar will remain elevated for a longer duration. This increases your risk for type 2 diabetes, cardiovascular disease, and cancer if it occurs frequently. By easily eating breakfast a little later and dinner a little earlier, it is possible to synchronize your food intake with your circadian rhythm and achieve an extended overnight fast without any additional effort.

Several studies have demonstrated that intermittent fasting improves cognition. Particularly, memory improvements have been discovered. There is evidence that intermittent fasting improves cognition, especially memory. It has been demonstrated that physical coordination and balance also improve alongside cognitive performance. Researchers are currently investigating the effects of intermittent fasting in areas where pharmacological treatments have failed, such as the progression of neurodegenerative diseases and physical challenges like frailty.

Intermittent fasting has been shown to be effective in treasily eating a variety of conditions that commonly affect the elderly, but its long-term efficacy is still being studied. Because the majority of research has focused on shorter time periods and the diet is difficult for some individuals to adhere to, little is known about the effects of time-restricted meals or calorie restriction on older individuals over the long term.

Some scientists wish to develop a pharmaceutical treatment that mimics the effects of intermittent fasting. Nevertheless, these techniques have not been shown to be as safe or effective as intermittent fasting. Due to intermittent fasting, a number of heart disease-related variables are reduced. The levels of high blood pressure, bad cholesterol, and triglycerides are examples. It can assist in cancer treatment. Intermittent fasting may have a positive effect on the prevention and treatment of cancer. Because cancer prevention research has been limited thus far, the word "may" is employed.

We have a connection with our body. Every time we breathe, our bodies communicate with us. We call it a stubbed toe when we touch our toe or burn our hand. Frequently, the messages are sent over a hot pan. It is brash, distinct, and rapid.

www.ingramcontent.com/pod-product-compliance
Lightning Source LLC
Chambersburg PA
CBHW050006070726
47592CB00018B/1066